The 1975 Pere Marquette
Theology Lecture

THE CONTRIBUTIONS
OF THEOLOGY
TO
MEDICAL ETHICS

by JAMES M. GUSTAFSON

University Professor of Theological Ethics
University of Chicago

Marquette Univerity Press
Milwaukee, Wisconsin 53233
April 6, 1975

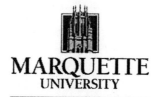

MARQUETTE
UNIVERSITY
PRESS

Second Printing 1977
Third Printing 1982
Fourth Printing 2001

© 1975, 2001
Marquette University Press
Milwaukee WI USA

ISBN 0-87462-507-6

MARQUETTE UNIVERSITY PRESS
MILWAUKEE

The Association of Jesuit University Presses

PREFACE

In conjunction with the Tercentenary Celebration of the missions and explorations of Jacques Marquette, S.J., the University's namesake, the Marquette University Theology Department in 1969 launched a series of annual public lectures by distinguished theologians under the title of "The Pere Marquette Theology Lectures."

The 1975 lecture was delivered at Marquette University on April 6, 1975, by Professor James M. Gustafson, University Professor of theological Ethics at the Divinity School of the University of Chicago.

Professor Gustafson was born in 1925 in Norway, Michigan. He completed his undergraduates studies at Northwestern University in 1948. In 1951 he received his B.D. from the federated Theological Faculty of the University of Chicago. In 1955 he received his Ph.D. from Yale University. Professor Gustafson is an ordained minister in the United Church of Christ.

Professor Gustafson is a widely known author and lecturer in the field of theological ethics. In addition to numerous articles, his major books include: *Treasure in Earthen Vessels* (1961), *Christ and the Moral Life* (1968), *The Church as Moral Decision Maker* (1970), *Christian Ethics and the Community* (1971), and *Theology and Christian Ethics* (1974). Professor Gustafson is the editor of *On Being Responsible: Issues in Personal Ethics* (1968) and co-author of *Advancement of Theological Education* (1956). His latest book, *Can Ethics Be Christian?*, has recently been published by the University of Chicago Press.

The present lecture reflects Professor Gustafson's long-standing interest in the area of medical ethics and his special concern for theology's proper contribution to this extremely complex field.

THE CONTRIBUTIONS OF THEOLOGY TO MEDICAL ETHICS

A person whose primary field of interest is theology can contribute to literature about ethics and medicine without articulating the theological grounds for the arguments and judgments that are made. When the theologian does so, he or she is functioning primarily as a moral philosopher, though as a philosopher who is working out of a particular theological moral point of view. To do so is not necessarily an act of deception, either of oneself or of others. Frequently the failure to develop the theological grounds for one's work in medical ethics stems from lack of interest in those grounds on the part of the particip-ants in the discussions of clinical moral issues. Frequently it stems from the effort to be persuasive on such grounds as diverse persons can agree upon; often to introduce theology becomes an unjustifiable reason for one's secular colleagues to discount what one might say about medical ethics.[1] The purpose of this lecture is to develop a position on the contribution that theology can make to medical ethics, attending both to the forms of the contribution and to the substance of it.

The order of development of the argument is as follows. First, it is necessary to indicate clearly what I mean when I speak of theology and of the work of a theologian, for different persons have different perceptions and convictions about what theology is. In a similar way, I shall indicate briefly what I think are the relevant dimensions of ethics. Second, theology is a source of many substantive themes which pertain to ethics, and to medical ethics particularly; I have isolated three affirmations to use illustratively in order to develop the more inclusive intention of this lecture. These are delineated and developed with reference to their contributions to a theological moral point of view, to certain relevant moral attitudes toward human life, and to a basic intentionality that informs action. In the course of the lecture, I indicate some of the ways in which the contribution of theology to medical ethics must be supplemented from other resources adequately to address particular clinical moral issues.

Theology and Ethics

Some clarification is required of the term "theology;" at least the way it is used here must be delineated. One distinction honored in the Christian tradition is between natural theology and revealed theology. I prefer not to use those two adjectives, for in the minds of historically and theologically learned or ecclesiastically contentious persons, they immediately indicate a debate that I seek to avoid. My view is stated in fewer words than desirable, but I hope with intelligibility.

I regard all of theology as reflection upon human experience; unfortunately in the Cristian community today there are those who think that statement is almost completely reversible; there are those who seem to regard all serious reflection on human experience as theology. Theology is reflection on human experience with reference to a particular dimension of the human experience denoted "religious." For many persons in the world of religion these days, any dimension of experience that is ultimate, integrative, or passionately felt, is "religious."[2] I distinguish my usage from such elastic references to the word religious. I reserve the word "religious" for that dimension of experience (in which not all persons consciously share) that senses a relationship to an ultimate power that sustains and stands over against humans and the world.[3] Thus, in this usage there is nothing properly called religion where there is no sense of the reality of an ultimate power, or of objective powers (to remember that there are polytheistic religions). The ultimate power is never experienced directly and immediately (perhaps an exception might be a rare experience of a rare mystic), but is always experienced indirectly and in a mediated way. Thus, to paraphrase John E.

Smith of Yale, an experience of the reality of God is always at one and the same time an experience of something else.[4] Alas, that statement is not convertible: an experience of an historical event, for example, is not necessarily a meaningful experience of God. Thus, to speak of the religious dimensions of experience is not to assert that every person is aware of such, or that persons who are aware of such are conscious of their significance in every experience they have. The oddity of religion lies in the fact that some persons do meaningfully and affectively experience an ultimate power sustaining and standing over against them. Sometimes this is in facing death, sometimes in eating a hot dog, sometimes in sequences of historical events, and sometimes in the voice of a friend.

Theology is an intellectual discipline that seeks to draw inferences (in a perhaps imprecise use of that term) from those dimensions of experience with reference to the power that is experienced. Thus, telling a story of a life experience is not itself theology, though there seems to be massive confusion on that point in the latest religious fad. Rather, a story is merely data for theological reflection. Theology seeks to determine, on the basis of inferences from the religious dimensions of experience, what qualities and characteristics can be appropriately attributed to the ultimate power, what purposes and intentions can be plausibly claimed for it, and what its relations are to the world. Philosophers with certain interests reflect upon the necessary conditions for anything to be, or on the necessary conditions for anything to be good, to be of value. The activities of such philosophers is similar to that of theologians and may assist them in their own task of drawing inferences by drawing in "transcendental deductions" or other procedures of thinking. But they are not necessarily doing theology. Theology takes place within the religious consciousness, or the experience and consciousness of the reality of God. Theology begins its task as a religious task. It is not the end result of any task that can be called an ontological or a methaphysical process of reflection.

What some persons call "revealed theology" I would prefer to call the theological reflection that occurs within a part of the human community whose experience of an ultimate power is nourished and informed by the most significant events, concepts and symbols, and by the historical continuities of life and thought of a particular tradition. It is not that only the Jewish or Christian communities experience the reality of God, or that their ways of articulating the purposes and attributes of God, and the modes of God's relations to the world, are the only valid ones. Indeed, they are historically conditioned, have often been partial, perhaps sometimes have been fundamentally mistaken. Historically, the Biblical peoples and their descendants have articulated inferences drawn from experience of the ultimate power as it has been known in many dimensions of life: in simply being alive itself, in the experience of betrayal and of trust, in life story of individuals, in political order and political chaos, in the sense of moral obligation and of moral values, in the experience of guilt and forgiveness, and many others. The narratives and the myths, the cryptic "I am who I am" and the fuller "I am the God of your father, the God of Abraham, the God of Isaac, and the God of Jacob,"[5] the laws and the prophetic utterances, the spiritual quarrels of Job and Jeremiah and the comforting assurances of benedictions and ascriptions to glory, the depictions of the special significance of Jesus in the writings of Paul, the authors of the Synoptic Gospels and John and others — all of these and others are articulations of a more general human experience of an ultimate power. Their "authority" for any time has a subjective dimension (it is not positivistic revelation); that dimension is a confirmation in the lives of persons that there is an authenticity and a validity in these articulations.

Thus, to be a Christian theologian is not to have a positivistic package of revealed theology, but to be one who reflects upon the reality of God experienced in and through many occasions of life in continuity with the history, the myths, the symbols and the concepts of people in that tradition. It is to draw inferences about the ultimate power, and to articulate them with confidence in, though not uncritical reliance upon, the articulations in the tradition. To be a Christian theologian, however, is not to be restricted to that tradition's literature as if it were the sufficient source for understanding all experience of the reality of God. The genus is theologian or theology; the species is Christian. When there are persuasive reasons for revising, altering, discarding, and adding to traditional articulations, it is the intellectual obligation of the theologian to do so.

In sum, I am using theology in a

restricted sense: it is the discipline in which finite and fallible human agents attempt to articulate in symbols, concepts and statements, the *logos*, the form and purposes of the ultimate power experienced in and through the experience of other things. On the basis of such articulations one can proceed to theological interpretations of many different events and objects, but that is another step.

From my perspective, ethics, like theology, is reflection on human experience. It is relection on human experience in its moral dimensions. The salient aspect of human experience in which moral dimensions occur is action. Ethics is an intellectual activity like theology. Its principal subject matter is human action. It is not all human action, however, but human action that is prescribed, governed, and judged by

moral values and by moral principles. The task of a moral philosopher
is two-fold: to analyze the necessary
conditions for moral activity (including moral judgments, and choices,
and actions) to occur, and to indicate
normatively what moral principles
and values ought to govern human
action. Ethics, like theology, is the
work of finite and fallible human
agents.

The *religious* qualification of
moral experience and more particularly of moral action, takes place
through the awareness that action
is not only in response to other persons, events, and things, but also in
response to the ultimate power that
sustains and stands over against
creation. Moral experience in the
context of religious life is qualified
affectively and intellectually by the
experience of the reality of God.[6] The
theological qualification of *ethics*

takes place through the articulation of the significance of the ultimate power both as a necessary condition for moral action, and as a necessary justification for moral values and principles that judge, prescribe, and govern action. The theologian who concentrates on ethics has the same two tasks as the moral philosopher: to analyze the necessary conditions for moral activity to occur, and to indicate normatively what moral principles and values ought to govern action. His difference from the moral philosopher is not in the *form* of thought, nor is the *substance* of this thought unique. His thought is qualified by his experience of and belief in the reality of God. Thus, his analysis of the necessary conditions for moral activity to occur will move to the theological margins of moral experience, and to the theological grounds of all experience. His indication of normative moral principles and values will be, in some manner, justified by his theology.

Medicine, I take it, merely specifies an arena of human action of which morality is a dimension. Thus medical ethics addresses this arena.

The Contribution of Theology to Medical Ethics

The contribution that theology can make to medical ethics depends upon what claims are made and defended about God, the ultimate power, and about human beings as moral agents in relation to God. Particularly it depends upon whether the symbols or concepts of God provide a basis for drawing moral inferences with reference to human activity. Moral inferences from theological claims have been made in many ways in the history of the Christian tradition. God has been claimed to be the giver of the moral law through persons such as Moses and through the moral order of creation via his gracious creative act.[7] God has been claimed to be the commander who speaks to people in a direct and immediate way in particular circumstances.[8] Stories and symbols of God and his activities have been used to interpret the religious and moral significance of events and circumstances in such a way that a particular course of human moral action "follows" from such interpretation.[9] "If a religious utterance is not a moral utterance no moral inferences can be drived from it . . . ."[10] In the Western religious traditions many "utterances" about God have moral terms.

The claims made about God that are bases for drawing moral infer-

ences, it must be noted, are not always straightforward predicates,
like "God is love," nor are they always general indicative statements,
like "God intends the well-being of
the creation." Often they have been
made in other forms of discourse,
God is like a King, or a Father, or a
Shepherd; analogies to social roles
imply certain relations, which in
turn are sources for delineating certain moral purposes or duties. God
chastizes his people for their religious and moral wrongs through the
activity of their political and milit-
ary enemies; culpability is punished
and thus the laws given to guide his
people are reinforced. God's rule is
like a Kingdom which will come;
from some perceptions of that Kingdom inferences are drawn about the
moral order that anticipates it. It is
not possible here to develop the var-
iety of religious language about God,

and to show how choices of significant symbols that refer to him and to
his activity richly affect the ways in
which the contributions of theology
to medical ethics can be made. God's
purposes, and his relations to creation about which Psalmists spoke
poetically, and prophets vividly,
must be indicated in briefer and
more prosaic terms.

To develop the contributions of
theology to medical ethics briefly, I
have selected three theological
themes to be used illustratively. In-
evitably this selection skews the
presentation, and invites possible
misinterpretations; yet in order to
indicate both in substance and in
form what the contribution of theology can be, it must be made. Two of
these themes are primarily about
God, one is primarily about humans.

First, God intends the well-being
of the creation. This statement

about God's intention clearly contains a value term, well-being. It is a declaration about God's purpose, or about what God values.

Second, God is both the ordering power that preserves and sustains the well-being of the creation and the power that creates new possibilities for well-being in events of nature and history. This theme is about the characteristic activities of the ultimate power. It also contains the value term, well-being. To use language more appropriate to humans, the first statement refers to the intention of God's "intellect" and the second to the intention of his "will" or "activity."

These statements about God, I believe, are plausible as inferences drawn from the religious dimensions of experience as that has been reflected upon by the Jewish and Christian communities, and expressed both in vivid symbols and in doctrinal statements. The experiences which make these symbolic and doctrinal affirmations plausible have been the occasions for the poetic and prayerful celebrations of the goodness of life in the tradition. The experiences which render them dubious have been the occasions for the most profound human quarrels with God, such as those of Job and Jeremiah, and for the elements of eschatological hope that are present in the tradition such as the expectation of a messiah, a return of the Lord, or the coming of God's Kingdom. "Philosophical" theologians have also on occasion found bases for making similar affirmations. I cannot here develop the grounds for plausibility of these statements; persons who find them plausible can follow the remainder of the argument with some conviction; persons who do not might follow it as a thought-experiment.[11]

The human race has developed in such a way that it has unique capacities among the whole of creation, namely those which enable its members to act intentionally to affect the course of the creation for its well-being. The human race has a role of "deputyship" or "stewardship" within creation. Humans are part of creation; they are finite. They are limited in information, understanding, and power, though in all three respects their capacities are beyond that of other creatures. In addition, distinctive human capacities are the conditions for a basic anxiety; human perceptions of life with its threats to individual and collective human well-being lead to inordinate efforts to secure and defend a time and space of stability to the cost of other persons and communities and other aspects of creation. Thus, relative to the ultimate power, God, humans are finite; relative to God's purpose and activity for the well-being of the whole of creation, humans are inordinately curved in upon their narrow self-interests in efforts to find security.[12] Our third statement sums this up. Humans are finite and "sinful" agents whose actions have a large measure of power to determine whether the well-being of the creation is sustained and fulfilled.

Whether the well-being of the creation will be preserved and sustained, and whether it will develop in response to events in history and nature that create new possibilities, depends to a large measure upon human action. Therein is built the principal bridge between theological beliefs and human morality. To reiterate, to determine whether well-being occurs, or whether something less than or opposite to it occurs, is in a large measure within the capacities of human agents. Medical research and practice is an arena in which finite and sinful humans have capacities to intervene in the biological processes of life in such a way that God's intention for the well-being of the creation is furthered or frustrated, in such a way that God's power to sustain and preserve that well-being is actualized or not, in such a way that the new possibilities that the creative power of God brings into being are fulfilled, partially realized, or turned to the devastation of the creation. The more precise arenas are many: clinical situations in which life can be prolonged, fetal life aborted, and disturbed patients committed to institutions; public health issues in which diseases can be controlled by pesticides, and resistance to illness developed by improvement in nutrition; medical research in which pharmacological means are developed to increase the stature of dwarfed humans or to control aggressive behavior, and genetic research in which inherited physical defects are isolated for potential therapy.

The issues that the argument must address can now be made more precise. What do these belief statements contribute to human moral action in the arena of medical practice and research? What do they contribute to an interpretation of the necessary conditions for moral action? What do they contribute to the establishment of moral principles and values which ought to be used to judge and guide action? How are these contributions made?

I shall proceed to develop the contributions in elaborations of each of the following proposals. 1. These beliefs contribute to medical ethics by providing a moral point of view, that is, a fundamental moral perspective on medical care and research. 2. These beliefs contribute to medical ethics by grounding and informing certain attitudes toward life which are significant for medical ethics. 3. These beliefs contribute to medical ethics by grounding and informing a basic ethical intentionality that gives direction to intervention in the biological processes of life.

Theology and a Moral Point of View

Theology contributes to medical ethics by providing a moral point of view. It provides a theological answer to the question, "Why be moral?" One ought to be moral because the ultimate power, God, intends (both in his "intellect" and in his "activity") that human actions conform to his purposes and activity for the well-being of the creation. Theology also provides some clues to human understanding of what the ultimate power values; a theological moral point of view not only answers the question, "Why be moral?" but also grounds some of the "substantive" bases for determining what values and principles ought to establish the point from which human action in the medical arena is morally directed and evaluated.[13] A theological moral point of view cannot claim to be unique in all of its aspects or dimensions; as it is delineated one sees that some of its aspects are present in views that eschew all references to theology.

To make clear some aspects of a theological moral point of view the first two themes particularly must be kept in mind. God intends the well-being of the creation. God is both the ordering power that preserves and sustains the well-being of the creation and the power that creates new possibilities for well-being in events of nature and history.

One characteristic of this moral point of view is its theological element in a most singular sense. God, the ultimate power, wills the well-being of creation; *God* orders its preservation and sustenance; *God* creates conditions for new possibilities of action. The implications of this need to be made explicit. Morality is not authorized merely by social conventions, though social conventions are necessary in the daily course of moral existence, and are often cited as a *prima facie* authority for both constraints and restraints upon action in medical care and research. Morality is not authorized merely by individual desires for human self-fulfillment, though the fundamental desire for human self-fulfillment is a significant motivating power for action on behalf of oneself and others. Morality is not authorized merely by the requirements of human rationality, though rationality has a crucial function in all of morality. From a theological point of view morality is authorized and required by God, the ultimate power.

For persons who participate in the religious outlook and consciousness of Biblically grounded religions this radically intensifies that seriousness of moral activity. Moral responsibilities and obligations are not only to the society or the profession to which one belong; they are not only to oneself and to other individuals; they are not only to the demands for rationality; they are responsibilities and obligations to God. Actions are judged to be wrong not only because of harms they cause to society, or to oneself and other individuals, or because they violate universal or general rules of conduct that reason demands. Actions are wrong because they violate the purposes and the activity of God, the ultimate power. This most distinctively theological aspect of a moral point of view characteristically marks persons whose moral action is carried out within a religious consciousness from persons who do not share in such an outlook. It most distinguishes the moral theologian from the secular moral philosopher.

A second characteristic of this moral point of view is its fundamental orientation toward the *well-being* of the creation. The import of this can be seen if a contrast is drawn with statements that the ultimate power is indifferent to values, or wills the destruction of the creation. If God were sheer power without "goodness," if he were being without value, a theological point of view would be a-moral, and theology could make no positive contribution to ethics. If the ultimate power willed the destruction of creation, there would be license not only for radical exploitation of life by humans in any given generation, but also for its utter demise. If God were indifferent to values, there would be no persistent moral thrust to human activity understood in a theological context; there would be no basic moral orientation to give direction and content to human activity. Since God wills well-being, the theological moral point of view is one which directs human action toward the realization of potentialities for value that are present in nature and in history.

A third characteristic is to be noted in my use of the well-being of *creation*. I have not stated that God wills the well-being exclusively of human individuals, or of human beings collectively. To be sure, it would not be proper to infer that the basic orientation of the ultimate power is antithetical to *human* well-being, but it is proper to suggest that the well-being of creation sets human well-being in a much wider context. One significance of this lies in the possibility that human perceptions of and convictions about what constitutes individual or communal well-being under particular conditions might be overridden by a concern for the "common good" of the whole creation. The concept of the "common good" has classically been limited to the good of the human community, or more characteristically to the good of particular communities such as a family or a nation. It has pointed toward the good of a community that is more than an aggregate or the sum of the goods of all its individual members. There are "goods" in proper relation of members to each other in the community; the common good is a relational and distributive concept. In affirming that God wills the well-being of the *creation* I propose an extension of the usage of the common good. It becomes necessary to think of the good of plants and water, air and minerals, as well as the good of human communities. It is necessary to think of the proper relations between humans and the rest of creation, of the proper distribution of "what is due" not only to persons but also to animals and plants. An act of moral imagination is required to extend the customary reference of the concept to the non-human world of which humankind is but a part.[14] If the "totality" (to use a term common to Roman Catholic moral theology) to be kept in view is extended from the physical body of a single individual to particular human communities, to the whole of the human community, and most inclusively to the whole of the creation, a basis has been established for the possibility that under certain conditions the well-being of a single individual, or even groups of persons might be overridden for the sake of the common good of the whole.[15] My intention is not to open the way for sweeping disregard for individual rights and claims to well-being, but to indicate that there might be a theological moral justification based on the common good of the creation for weighing the "value" of the whole in relation to the "value" of

individual humans, or to that of particular values to which particular
human groups cleave as necessary
for their "well-being."

Another significance of "the
well-being of the *creation*" is that it
requires a subordination of human
ends as those that all of the rest of
creation serves. This is an alteration
of a view that has been strongly present in Western religion and morality. While there are no grounds for
denying that in a descriptive sense
the human race has developed to
heights of capacities and achievements beyond that of any other
creatures on earth, such a "natural
hierarchy" can be endowed with a
hierarchy of value that exalts the
distinctive value of the human to the
detriment of the creation of which
the human is but a part. Humankind, by virtue of its capacities,
clearly has a distinctive role within

the life of the creation; its natural abilities extended through culture give it distinctive responsibilities as well as distinctive possibilities for well-being. But a simplistic equation of a hierarchy of beings with a hierarchy of values, and a heedless equation of the well-being of the human with values of immediate self-interest can be questioned on the grounds of the affirmation that God intends the well-being of the *creation*. Judgments are possible from this theological moral point of view which override certain human claims for individual rights and values for the sake of the more inclusive well-being of a wider circle of life. Circumstances have arisen in which the right to unlimited human procreation, for example, is a threat to the well-being of the whole creation. Other circumstances are conceivable in which the preservation of individual physical lives might be judged to be a threat to the well-being of the whole.[16]

A fourth characteristic of the moral point of view developed from the first two theological themes is that they ground principles for the conservation and preservation of life. Wherever and whenever the well-being of the creation is threatened, and particularly the well-being of human physical life as the condition *sine qua non* for all other forms of human well-being, there is a basis for critical moral indictment. That God is an ordering power whose presence and activity seeks to preserve and sustain life leads to principles that are essentially conservative in their function. The known and experienced values of life, and particularly of human life, are not to be overridden without exceptionally good moral reasons.

Intrusions into individual lives, or into the course of biological development, that are likely to be both destructive and irreversible cannot be undertaken without exceptionally strong justifications. Clear moral indictments are called for whenever conditions occur in which the well-being of creation is threatened, whether that be indiscriminate use of the weapons of warfare, the lack of proper nourishment for families or for whole populations, the lack of adequate health-care when capacities for such are available, or heedless actions that are deleterious to the well-being of persons and their social and natural environments.

The fifth characteristic is that these theological themes provide a basis for the alteration of principles articulated from past traditions and experiences, for the extension and revision of principles and values that have traditionally been adhered to in medical research and care. It provides a basis for a re-ordering of accepted values in the light of new conditions when there is warrant for such. God not only acts to sustain and preserve life, but his power creates the conditions in which new possibilities for well-being occur, and in which different actions are required to preserve the well-being of the whole of creation. This characteristic of the theological moral point of view I am developing here requires more extensive discussion, for I believe it distinguishes my thought from that of some other theologians, and is also the most controversial aspect of it.

Certainly it distinguishes it from the manuals of traditional Roman Catholic moral theology on medical questions.[17] The distinction is based on a theological conviction that makes a moral difference. The authors of the traditional manuals tend to view the principles of well-being of both humans and the rest of creation as fixed and immutable; God established a moral order in creation. He was not so much, as he is in my view, creating in nature, history, and culture possibilities for different patterns of well-being. Thus the ethics grounded in the theology of natural law that was regnant until recently have been consistently very conservative with reference to medical research and practice. They have been an ethics of preservation of life that admirably led to restraints of actions which were costly for individuals and often for societies. On the basis of their versions of natural law Catholic moralists provided what were in fact formidable dikes against morally heedless actions. Restraints which have preserved individual well-being of present persons, however, have perhaps sometimes led to neglect of justifiable benefits and created harms for more inclusive communities of persons, and have possibly been deleterious to future generations.[18]

This characteristic distinguishes my view from that of my Protestant theological colleague, Paul Ramsey. In Ramsey's theology the central ethical principle is love, *agapé*. Its source is the Scriptures. *Agapé* must be "in-principled" in order to be applicable to disparate human circumstances such as the conduct of warfare and medical care and research. In Ramsey's "in-principling" of love he chooses to develop Christian ethics as deontological ethics, ethics of obligation and duty governed by principles and rules, rather than dominantly as ethics of value or ends. "Certainly Christian ethics is a deontological ethic, not an ethic of 'the good'."[19] Love is not developed primarily as a motive term, as it frequently is in Christian ethics. Ramsey has good reasons with which I agree for not attending to love as a motive as the principal reference of the term and the reality; to do so often does not provide clear principles for discriminating between the rightness and wrongness of actions, all of which can claim to be motivated by love. Nor is love developed primarily as a value term, as a term that can be used to order the relative values of certain potential ends or consequences of medical and other actions. Ramsey's good reasons for eschewing this tack are those that all critics of utilitarian ethics make: consequences are not fully predictable; consequences are not commensurable in the way that "cost-benefit" analysis strives to make them; the criteria for evaluating benefits and harms are extraordinarily slippery, and so forth.[20] I share Ramsey's critical analysis of simple utilitarianism. Love becomes, for Ramsey, basically a concept of human fidelity, and is reinforced by the notions of "covenant fidelity" that are grounded in the Old Testament. Physicians have obligations of fidelity to patients by virtue of the "contract" that is established between them, and the primary substance of these obligations is to act in the best interests of the individual patients. Obviously some consideration of consequences is required to determine those interests, and the first rule in judging those consequences for Ramsey is "Do no harm." In effect, "Do no harm" and especially "Do no harm to those who cannot consent to an intrusion" becomes a rule which physicians and investigators have an absolute obligation to obey.[21] This is an example of deontological ethics derived from *agapé* with reference to medical practice.

Just as theological differences distinguish my position from that of the authors of traditional Roman Catholic texts on medical moral theology, so there are theological differences between Ramsey and me. I believe there would be little difference between us on the significance of the third theme I stated above, that which pertains to the finitude and sinfulness of human agents. Nor would there be a significant difference on the first part of the second theme, that which pertains to sustenance and preservation of well-being. Unlike the Roman Catholics alluded to, Ramsey does not have a theory of natural law as a basis for his ethics, though he freely borrows concepts from the tradition in executing his deontological ethics. His conservative judgments on medical research and care are derived, in distinction from theirs, from his view of *agapé* and covenant fidelity between persons. In practice this becomes largely fidelity to known obligations and is done to sustain known benefits for individuals. The crucial theological difference between Ramsey and me is in the emphasis that I give to God as the power that creates new possibilities for well-being in events of nature and history, including the possibilities that emerge in the course of evolutionary development and the development of biological knowledge. This emphasis opens ethically the possibilities for an alteration of some traditional princi-

ples, and an alteration of the ordering of certain traditional values in
particular circumstances.

Random and heedless experimentation with human life is fenced by
principles inferred from God's preservative activity and from the finite and sinful human condition.
Thus there are no grounds for a
license to engage in therapeutic or
other forms of experimentation
without careful rational discrimina-
tion between possible harmful and
beneficial consequences to individual persons, to the human community and to the whole of creation.
But neither is human physical life of
absolute value; God wills the well-
being of the *creation*. Just as there
are historical occasions on which
human physical life is not only
risked but sacrificed for what is
judged to be a human common good,
for example, in the defense of a na-

tion against unjust attack, so also there are occasions in which new possibilities for the well-being of individual persons, the human community, and the whole of creation require action that risks harm, indeed, irreversible harm, to individuals. Known benefits must be risked for unknown; known harms can sometimes be avoided only by risking known benefits. Action is by finite human agents; it is inherently risky and frequently unavoidably tragic in the strongest sense. The creation of new possibilities by the ultimate power has throughout the whole of evolutionary and cultural development been costly to many species of life, and to valued human achievements. There is no avoidance of ambiguity, and there is also no excuse for failure to reason carefully about intrusions into human life that become possible. There is no guarantee that development is moral progress, but there is also no guarantee that restraints upon action by a deontological principle "Do no harm" to a particular individual or species fulfills the well-being of the creation.[22]

The theological moral point of view developed here has some things in common with that being developed by Professor Karl Rahner. In his article, "Experiment with Man," for example, Father Rahner compacts his philosophical anthropology and his theology into a basis for a cautious argument against those persons who would be unduly restrictive about experimentation with human beings. Toward the end of the article he writes,

One ought soberly and courageously to consider, according to a supra-individual morality, what sacrifices could be expected of humanity today on behalf of humanity tomorrow, *without* being too quick to speak of immoral cruelty, of the violation and exploitation of the dignity of man today for the benefit of man tomorrow.[23]

He invokes theologically a basis for a moral realism within the context of hope so that "the Christian has no reason to enter this future as a hell on Earth nor as an earthly Kingdom of God."[24] "Christianity," he avers, "is the religion of the absolute future to the extent in the first place that God is not only 'above us' as the ground and horizon of history, but 'in front of us' as our own future, our destination, sustaining history as its future."[25] He also reminds us that "self-manipulation and all its concrete and utopian aims are constantly subject to the law of death— which can be neither disposed of nor manipulated."[26] But more crucial for his argument is his philosophical and theological anthropology. The distinction between the human dimension of "fundamental transcendental freedom" and the capacities for "categorial self-manipulation" must be understood in order to comprehend the openness to change and the caution that are involved in Rahner's moral point of view. Stated oversimply, Rahner locates the distinctively human in man's transcendental freedom; this freedom, which is radical, is always categorially situated in bodily and historical existence. Human actions which actualize the capacity for personhood, for freedom, are desirable. What actualizes this capacity, however, is discovered in part by human "self-manipulation" through the course of human experience and there are still things to be discovered. Human "nature" is not immutable; human knowledge is not complete. In this lies the warrant for greater openness to experimentation than traditionalistic Catholics permit. Yet his own negative judgment (with which I disagree) about artificial insemination by a non-husband donor in "The Problem of Genetic Manipulation" indicates that Rahner does not give license for heedless intrusions into human biological life. Thus Rahner derives from his anthropology preservative principles, but also a basis for taking risks to discover what fulfills the human spirit in the course of human experience.[27]

To sort out the differences between the proposal I am making and Rahner's theology and philosophical anthropology is far too intricate and extensive a task to be undertaken here. It will have to suffice to indicate that Rahner's guarded openness to experimentation with humans is grounded primarily in his anthropology, whereas the theological theme from which mine is derived is that God is creating conditions for new possibilities of well-being in the creation. Also, in spite of Rahner's invocation of a "supra-individual morality," in my judgment his focus remains too exclusively on humans, and has excessively individualistic tendencies. Just as it is not easy to develop a social ethics for institutions and politics from Rahner's work, so also it is difficult to see how one would develop an ethics that would extend the concept of the "common good" to include the whole creation. Overtones of an inordinate value to the human remain in Rahner's work. Nonetheless, as James F. Bresnahan has amply demonstrated, Rahner's theology and philosophy provide a basis for a developmental view of human understanding of what the "natural law" requires.

Human "self-manipulation" is not only a datum of history and culture, but is grounded in the essence of the human.[28]

In summary, the fifth characteristic of the theological moral point of view developed here takes a process of natural and historical development to be more central as a basis for medical ethics than do some other theological views. To use the notion of humans as "co-creators" with God is too strong; to view God as creating conditions for new possibilities to which humans respond, however is proper. Perhaps the term "co-actors" is appropriate. Human actions are responsive to and responsible to the ultimate power that brings different conditions into being. Because there is continuity in the purposes and activities of God, there are not sufficient grounds for judging that the new conditions require a radically "new morality." Because new possibilities develop both naturally and as a result of human knowledge and interventions into biological life, it is not always possible to be responsible for the well-being of the creation and at the same time to preserve certain rights of individuals that in the past were judged inalienable. It is sometimes morally justifiable to alter the order of values from the past in the light of different and novel conditions.

Some of the well-being that our present life in creation provides has been very costly to species of animals and plants, some of which were extinct long before the emergence of our species. This continues to be the case. There is no guarantee that the future well-being of the creation can be protected without severe pain and cost to individual persons and even to particular communities. To insure and realize well-being for the creation (including humans as part of it) may require risks that incur irreversible deleterious consequences for some persons. This does not license innovative exploration for the sake of mere curiosity; a theological moral point of view presumes the priority of preservation. But from my theological perspective there must be an openness to the possibility of extending, or even altering, traditional moral principles and re-ordering traditional human values.

Theology and Attitudes

The three theological themes stated above contribute to the morality of medical research and care by grounding and informing certain attitudes toward biological life and toward medical activity. Attitudes: the plural is deliberate. Even the selection of only three theological themes indicates that several attitudes are grounded in Christian and Jewish religious beliefs. If God were asserted to be only the creative power that makes for novelty and new possibilities of action, a single attitude might be appropriate, namely one of "openness" to novelty, to "co-creative" activity with God. Such an attitude or disposition could be acted out in massive interventions within the given possibilities in medical research and practice. It might find expression in a maxim, "What can be done ought to be done." If God were only a preserving power, another single attitude would be grounded and informed, namely one of restraint. Persons with exclusively this attitude would be extraordinarily conservative; for the sake of preserving life as it is presently known and valued they would be unwilling to bear the risks required to extend human knowledge and enlarge the range of human action. The more "unitarian" one's view of God's purposes and activity is, the simpler are the attitudes that such an experience and conviction grounds and informs.[29] The theological themes I have selected ground several attitudes or dispositions. Three are developed here.

The condition *sine qua non* for well-being is the existence of life itself. From a theological perspective that views life as being created and sustained by an ultimate power who intends its well-being, a fundamental *attitude of respect for life* is evoked, grounded, and informed. Indeed, in the experience of the Biblical religious communities life is received from God; it is received from the ultimate power who creates, sustains and preserves it, and who creates new possibilities for well-being. It is received as the necessary condition for any value, any well-being, and thus is received as a value, as a good, and thus deserves respect. Thus the history of morality in the Western religions is hinged upon not only respect for what is not in the power of humans to create, but also on gratitude for life.[30]

Karl Barth, in a discussion that has received less attention than it ought to (probably because it is cast in his particular theological framework) reminds us that respect for life is to be directed toward all living things, plants and animals as well as humans.

> ... The world of animals and plants forms the indispensable living background to the living-space divinely allotted to man and placed under his con-

trol. As they live, so can he. He is not set up as lord over the earth, but as lord on the earth which is already furnished with these creatures. Animals and plants do not belong to him; they and the whole earth can belong only to God.[31]

An attitude of respect for life inhibits the drive to proprietary claims to exploit animals and plants, and even rocks and minerals, solely for the satisfaction of immediate interests of humans who have the capacities and the power to do so. While Albert Schweitzer's "reverence for life" appears to be tinged with a biological romanticism, it nonetheless points to the same limitations on human interventions. One implication of this attitude of respect can be seen in Barth's discussion of the slaying of animals.

The slaying of animals is really possible only as an appeal to God's reconciling grace . . . It undoubtedly means making use of the offering of an alien and innocent victim and claiming its life for ours. Man must have good reasons for seriously making such a claim.[32]

In the religious consciousness, our theological themes evoke the attitude of respect. This respect, as we have seen, is not due only to human physical life; it is due to the whole of creation. To have respect for the creation tempers destructive intrusions into all of life; it evokes a sense of accountability for all of creation; it leads to the requirement that good reasons must be given to intervene in the processes of biological life; it stimulates a note of anguish at the costs that are involved to the natural world for the sake of human comfort and well-being . Conflicts of values are not resolved by such an attitude of respect. Nature is not only a supportive "indispensable living background" to human life; it is frequently the enemy of humans.

Cancerous growths and cyclones, Arctic climates and destruction by beasts have all led to technologies to protect humans from the threats of nature. In medical care and research these conflicts take a particular form. For example, respect for life does not necessarily indicate the preservation of human physical life at the cost of unbearable pain to individuals, and even to families around them. Nonetheless, an attitude of respect is primary, for life is received from a power that wills its well-being.

"Life is no second God, and therefore the respect due to it cannot rival the reverence owed to God."[33] In this statement Barth indicates that respect for life does not entail an idolatrous reverence. This also is important to note. There are occasions in which the almost absolute value of physical life is justifiably sacrificed for other values. In the religious traditions of the west this has been more frequently affirmed with reference to social values such as justice or a nation's right to self-defense than with reference to intrusions in individual bodily life. One principle that has justified the taking of human life is the culpability of those who create unjust and repressive conditions, or who instigate an unjust attack on a nation. The insistence that there be a "just cause" for any sacrifice of human life has upheld a strong wall against inhumane destruction of individuals and groups. Nazi experimentation with humans, for example, is properly judged to be immoral not only because the subjects were judged to belong to a class of persons without basic human rights, but also because the importance of the knowledge gained was disproportionate with the costs. Moral restrictions on abortions have been established on the basis of the absence of a "just cause" to take innocent life. I recognize that to defend an attitude of respect for life while at the same time not giving human physical life absolute value is to place moral choices on a slippery slope. This difficulty clearly indicates that an attitude or a disposition is not sufficient to determine what a proper course of action ought to be. Additional ethical reflection is required to make particular moral judgments about, and to give moral direction to, interventions in biological life, both human and non-human. An attitude of respect for the creation does not in itself resolve the questions of what constitutes the well-being of creation in a particular time and place, nor does it univocally determine whose well-being is to be restricted or sacrificed for the well-being of other persons or of plants and air. There is no guarantee, however, of a cost-free or even risk-free way of making such determinations.[34]

If an attitude of respect for life is basically an inhibiting and conservative one (though under certain circumstance it might lead to radical interventions,[35]) the theme pertaining to God's creative power to develop new opportunities establishes an *attitude of "openness."* Since the grounds for this were developed extensively in the fifth characteristic of the theological moral point of view, it can be treated more briefly here. The attitude of openness coexists with the attitude of respect; whereas respect curbs openness from becoming a license for heedless interventions and explorations, openness keeps respect from becoming dogmatic and idolatrous.

Openness to new possibilities, or at least to different possibilities of action, has been present in extreme situations throughout the development of morality. Classic situations of triage have occurred where scarce resources are present and the demands upon the far more extensive than can be met. Justifications have been made for determining who shall have access to them on the basis of relative probabilities for survival.[36] Some persons have been permitted to die so that others have a greater possibility for life. Persons have survived apparently as a result of their willingness to eat human flesh in drastic circumstances. Indeed, physical survival appears to be an end that overrides all others in the most desperate circumstances.[37] The most extreme circumstances permit possible justification of an extension or alteration of traditional principles and of the ordering of values.

Openness, with an attendant courage to take risks, is warranted, I believe, in more than extreme survival situations. In instances in which openness has led to the improvement of grains and livestock through "manipulation" of what has been given by natural developments, the attitude and its fruits are lauded. Respect for persons is different in character from the respect due to plants and animals if only because of a primitive feeling of cohumanity that resists turning persons into means rather than ends, that resists the thingification of human beings and the purely technocratic consequences of such a choice.[38] There is a qualitative distinction between human life and other species that grounds a distinction in valuation, though, as I have argued, that value distinction has frequently been exaggerated. Thus to suggest that openness and courage to risk is appropriate to other than extreme situations is not to argue for "human engineering," or for the right of those who have knowledge and power to engage in radical medical experimentation without good moral reasons. It is, however, to suggest that there are justifications for risking serious costs to some persons for the sake of relieving their own suffering, and the suffering of others.

As with respect for life, so the openness to new possibilities is not sufficient as a basis for the ethics of human intervention, experimentally or therapeutically. The attitude must be supplemented by principles which, for example, insure the informed consent of persons who take risks. The reasonable intent of all experimentation involving severe risk must be demonstrably warranted by significant potential contributions to the well-being of humans. The theological grounding of this attitude is the affirmation that new possibilities emerge in the biological, historical, and cultural development of the creation as these are empowered by the creative activity of God. The failure to be responsive to such new possibilities, an absence of openness and courage, can lead to deleterious consequences via omission; this must always be recalled by those whose attitude is solely one of conservation of present well-being.[39]

The third attitude is one of *self-criticism*. This is particularly grounded in and informed by the third theological theme formulated above: humans are finite and "sinful" agents whose actions have a large measure of power to determine whether the well-being of creation is sustained and fulfilled.[40]

Recognition of finitude and its consequences comes through both the normal and the critical courses of human experience. Death is one inexorable indication of it. The crisis of scarcity of food and of energy that the world is currently realizing is another. Humans are finite agents: they cannot foresee all the consequences of their interventions into nature; they do not fully comprehend as yet all of the causal relationships between intended benefits of their interventions and unintended harmful consequences; they have, for all the powers of culture and technology have given them, limited capacities to control the effects of their actions. Human actions take place in a finite world of limited resources. While the marvelous capacities of the human brain and of culture develop new resources for life, there is no guarantee that in some future time the given resources will not be exhausted. The recognition of finitude evokes an attitude of self-criticism of choices and actions. We are created; we are not God.

This attitude is religiously and morally fitting in the arenas of medical care and research as well. To acknowledge human limitation is to be cautious about intrusions into individual bodies which might have destructive irreversible consequences. It is to be cautious about genetic research of certain sorts because of possible hazards to society.[41] It is to recognize that intervention into the human brain by surgery can cause deterioration of valued human capacities which cannot be renewed. It is to be aware that the best possible information and understanding is required before novel therapies and research on human and animal subjects is engaged in. Attitude, again, is not sufficient to determine what ought and ought not to be done in particular circumstances; a self-critical attitude needs supplementation of moral reflection about the principles and values that can give guidance to human interventions. The recognition of human finitude, and the self-critical attitude it grounds and informs, however, are indispensable to responsible medical practice.

From a theological perspective the human condition is not only one of finitude, but also one of sin. There is a profound tendency in humans to secure narrow self-interests and the interests of particular communities at the cost of the well-being of others. In Christianity this tendency is interpreted as a religious problem as well as a moral problem. It has been interpreted as a human effort to overcome the conditions of finitude by securing a basis of value and meaning for an individual or a community that functions as its god. In this striving for a ground of certitude there are almost inexorable consequences of exercising overweening power over others, and of depriving others of resources that are justly theirs. Among the forms that sin takes, pride is perhaps the most harmful in the area of medical care and research. The recognition of a sinful condition evokes an attitude of self-criticism, for it cautions human agents against insensitivity and blindness to their overweening desires for individual self-fulfillment or for the fulfillment of their professional or other communities by ignoring their obligations to others and engaging in actions which are costly to others. That an attitude of self-criticism is appropriate for "sinful" persons engaged in medical care and research needs no further explication or illustration.

In relation to the conditions of finitude and sin, one other aspect of moral experience needs to be noted which also sustains a self-critical attitude, namely the absence of absolute certitude about moral judgments, choices and actions. This does not imply that there are not varying degrees of certitude about the propriety of various moral principles and human values. The alternative to absolute certitude is not absolute relativism in medical ethics. Nor does it indicate that the moral wisdom accrued through the history of our culture is without authority or cannot be justified rationally. It is, however, to argue that with reference to some instances of clinical moral decisions and some instances of proposed medical experimentation agents are deprived of both absolute subjective and objective certitude that their actions are unambiguously right and good. If the moral act of the physician or investigator is judged purely with reference to his or her intention, greater claims for certitude can be made. If, however, the basis for determining whether a medical intervention is morally right or good involves also an assessment of its consequences both to the primary parties involved and to the society and the rest of creation, certitude is more difficult to secure. In addition to the conditions of finitude and sin, the developmental character of nature and society also necessitates a degree of uncertainty. If absolute certitude is not possible in certain circumstances, then an attitude of self-criticism is required.[42]

The attitudes of respect for life, of openness, and of self-criticism co-exist; as has been indicated, no single attitude is grounded in and informed by theological themes if those themes are properly inclusive. As illustrations of how theology contributes to the morality of medicine, they provide a pattern by which other attitudes can also be seen to be appropriate. No doubt different individuals in medical practice have different dominant attitudes; there are those who are more open to take risks in therapy and investigation, and those whose respect for life or whose self-criticism places restraint on their practice. One can note that communities of discourse in medical research and care are necessary for mutual correction and instruction.

The enterprise of medicine, while frequently practiced by isolated individuals, is a communal one, and the formation of attitudes takes place within professional communities.

As has also been noted, attitudes are not a sufficient basis for determining courses of action, or for making judgments about medical interventions. Tendencies to act in certain ways follow from persistent attitudes, but moral reflection of a more rational sort is also required both to check excessive reliance upon attitudes and to give specific direction to the actions toward which attitudes pre-dispose physicians and investigators.

Theology and Ethical Intentionality

Theological themes ground and inform a basic ethical intentionality that gives direction to action. The "substance" of that intentionality is that the well-being of the creation is to be sustained, preserved, and developed. The form must also be noted; it is a basic or general intentionality, and not a set of precise action-guiding rules or principles for critical evaluation of particular actions. To affirm that God intends the well-being of the creation is not a sufficient basis for medical ethics. To determine what constitutes that well-being, what is to be valued about both human life and the rest of creation, what principles, rights and obligations are to be adhered to in sustaining and developing well-being, requires many more sources than theology; certainly more than the themes chosen for this lecture.

The theological themes are basically teleological; they state an end that the ultimate power intends, and thus an end that is proper to human activity which is responsible to God. But the *telos* in such ethics must be defined or specified, and the options for doing this are several. Frequently the *telos* has been formulated in general terms. The end that humans seek as an end in itself, Aristotle wrote, is *eudaimonia*, usually translated "happiness." In the classic theology of Roman Catholicism, beings are created with a natural tendency toward their proper end, toward their "good." The overarching normative objective of classic utilitarianism is "the greatest good for the greatest number." The ambiguity of each of these statements has been noted often, for each requires more extensive elaboration of what constitutes human happiness, or the good that is the proper end of man, or the good that the greatest number ought to have. When the well-being of the whole of creation is the purpose of God, the difficulties of defining the "good" are compounded, for one must consider what is good for plants, water, animals and air as well as what is good for humans; and consideration must be given to the proper relations of these to each other for the "common good" of the creation. Clearly there are many "goods" or many values that constitute the well-being of the whole of creation.

The specification of the well-being of creation will yield a plurality of ends, or of values. This is also the case with reference to the well-being of individual persons and of human communities. The preservation of physical life is a good, but so is relief from unbearable or unrelievable physical pain in the process of dying. In the most classic of all dilemmas of medical care, the relief of pain and the preservation ·of physical life cannot be fulfilled together in every instance; either a choice must be made between conflicting ends, or a rationale given in which the proper moral intention to relieve pain has as an unintended consequence the death of the patient. A foreseeable benefit for other persons that will relieve them from disabilities of ill-nesses might be actualized only at the risk of some harm to persons who are the subjects of pertinent ex-perimentation. There is no automa-tic harmony in the immediacies of experience between the well-being of both the experimental subject and other persons. On the massive, non-medical scale of interventions into biological life there are many examples of interventions to relieve one impediment or harm only at the risk of unintended and even un-

foreseeable deleterious consequences for the ordering of nature.
The introduction of DDT is an example of this.

A less distinctively theological
task of ethics must be undertaken to
determine more precisely what constitutes well-being, and in the arena
of medicine, the well-being of individual persons and of human communities. There are several ethical
theories; beyond a basically teleological framework, the theological
principles used here do not in themselves determine which ethical
theory is necessary to develop the
ethics of medical care and research
in greater detail. Within a basically
teleological framework in which the
well-being of the creation is the end
or *telos*, it is possible to develop
ethics that are utilitarian in form,
such as Joseph Fletcher's well-
known "situation ethics."[43] But such

an ethical theory is not the necessary implication of the framework. It is possible to develop ethics similar to classic natural law ethics. It is possible to develop an ethics of principles and rules, and even an ethics that is deontological in its practical impact.

As John Rawls has noted, there is a two-step process involved in working out an ethics of rules.[44] One is to give reasons for the rules or principles; this justification can be utilitarian, or teleological, or something else. The moral rules pertaining to medical care and research can be justified, for example, on the grounds that they serve the well-being of the patients. The second step is the justification of particular actions under the rules or principles. For example, once a rule against overt euthanasia is justified as being in the best interests of all patients, there is a *prima facie* obligation to follow the rule; the physician does not have to support his response to each patient by giving reasons for the rule against overt euthanasia. But he must apply the rule to the circumstances of a particular patient. If he chooses to make an exception to the rule there must be unusually good reasons for doing so. In the case of an exception to the rule against euthanasia, no doubt the reasons would primarily be that the exception best fulfills the reason for the rule, namely that it is in the best interests of the patient. Within a teleologically justified system of rules for medical ethics, moralists can develop universal and unexceptionable rules, "general rules," or "summary rules." Certain actions might be judged to be intrinsically evil; they violate the essence of humanity, or what is essentially valued about humanity. An unexceptionable rule prohibiting such actions would follow.

Even a theologian who seeks to work out ethics from a Biblical confessional theology gives mixed ethical arguments to direct conduct in the medical arena. Karl Barth has developed an ethics of the commands of God. The proper human response to a command is obedience; thus moral action is proper when it is in obedience to the command of God. In Barth's ethics God commands a particular agent in particular circumstances. Yet, as Barth works out his practical ethics, it is clear that God's particular commands can be rationally justified. They will be in accord with his revelation in Jesus Christ and thus be reasonably coherent with Christological doctrines. In his "practical casuistry he also states rather distinctively ethical reasons pertaining to human rights and human ends with which God's commands are likely to concur. Barth's ethics, in form and vocabulary, are coherent with the Biblical theology that he develops. While God gives specific commands on each occasion, he is not capricious; thus his commands are likely to be consistent with the Decalogue and the Sermon on the Mount. Taken out of the theological context, this works out to be an ethics of general rules to which there might be exceptions on particular occasions. Thus abortion is judged to be morally wrong, but there are situations of conflict between fetal and maternal life in which an abortion is right. God can command it. It remains a sin, but it is a forgivable sin.[45] Euthanasia seems less likely to be commanded by God; his argument is supported by ethical reasons.

Medical ethics that are developed in relation to the theological themes used in this lecture, or from other theologies, necessarily use non-theological principles for their explication. The well-being of the creation cannot be defined by theological referents alone. Theology alone is not a sufficient basis for defining the human values and developing the moral rules and principles that are used to judge and to guide action in a particular arena like medical research and care. While the different ethical theories can be used to develop our theological themes there is a way of "doing ethics" which I believe is more appropriate to them than are others. It can be briefly developed.

The most important ethical task is to develop as precisely and thoroughly as possible the qualities of well-being — in medical research and care, those qualities that are valued about human physical life as the condition *sine qua non* for other values are of particular significance. This task involves not only an "empirical" dimension, that is, a determination of what is actually valued about human life, but also an ethical one. It requires a determination of what *ought* to be valued about human physical life and wide human experience, and giving grounds for answers to that *ought* question. What ought to be valued for the sake of human well-being yields a plurality of values: physical health, relief from avoidable suffering, and many more. Physical life is the condition *sine qua non* for all other values of human life; thus there is always a presumption in favor of sustaining it, or in favor of research that will yield knowledge which will aid in its sustenance. But physical life is not of absolute value.

The primary practical questions in medical research and care involve *conflicts of values*. Conflicts are inevitable because of the plurality of qualities that constitute human well-being; conflicts become more complex when the well-being of individuals is considered in relation to that of other persons, of human communities, and of the whole of creation. Only at a high level of ideational generalization can these conflicts be resolved. In particular circumstances of medical care and research there are sometimes choices that are inherently tragic in their consequences: to preserve one life is not to have the resources available to preserve the lives of others; to relieve parents of the anguish involved in caring for a child with the incurable and fatal Tay-Sachs disease requires that the life of the afflicted fetus be taken.

Since the inexorable conflicts of values usually are not unprecedented, or since there have been at least analogous conflicts in the past, it is not necessary to "re-invent the wheel" on each occasion. Since there is a heritage of ethical thought extending back to the early recorded history of the species, and since careful reflection has been given to the proper ordering of values, to the formulation of principles and rules for guiding action in circumstances of conflict, the medical profession has recourse to ethical ideas to guide its interventions procedurally and substantively. From previous experience and previous thought, various rules have been developed which presumptively ought to be obeyed, for they have led to the sustenance of human well-being, and to new resources that have been beneficial to humans. In routine matters, little or no further thought is required on the part of the agent beyond perception of what moral rules govern the class of circumstances to which an individual case belongs. Where conflicts are somewhat critical, general rules have been developed which can be violated only by giving good reasons that the case at hand is an exception. That exception will be justified by a rational assessment of which values *in the context of the relationships involved in that particular case* are most important.

In circumstances of great novelty, in which procedures of therapy or experimentation appear to be possible for which there are no significant precedents, the weighing of the values in conflict is more difficult, particularly if a proposed course of action has irreversible deleterious consequences for persons. Risk is greater. Rational certitude about the right course of action is more elusive. Analogies must be explored; general rules or principles applied insofar as possible and exceptions to them thought through carefully; probabilities of consequences must be weighed. No reasonably unexceptionable conclusion from a moral standpoint is possible in some such instances, though to fail to seek for such is irresponsible. I believe it is coherent with the three theological principles stated above to act in such circumstances if there appears to be a significant series of good reasons to do so, or if there are not good reasons for refraining from action. Absolute moral certitude, however, is impossible.

To be human is to be finite, and such certitude as God might have is not available to humans. Yet humans are responsible co-actors, or interactors with God whose purpose and activity can never be perfectly disclosed to finite creatures. The conditions of creatureliness necessitate risk; well-being might be diminished by inaction as well as by action. Further, as the creative power of God creates new possibilities for development of the human species and the rest of the creation, the process of discovering what constitutes well-being continues. Well-being is also, at least in some of its aspects, *relational;* its particular forms alter in relation to many natural and cultural factors. Health, for example, has different significance when used with reference to an adolescent from what it has with reference to an octogenarian. The discernment of what constitutes well-being is made in the course of alterations in the natural world and of human cultures. Certainly the possibility to realize particular aspects of well-being depends on the presence of particular relationships.

Finally, it must be noted that in the development of medical ethics within a theological perspective, the contributions of therapists and investigators are indispensable. Particular value conflicts occur in relation to courses of action that have definite characteristics. For example, if the moral theologian is to make judgments or to give moral counsel he or she must learn from medical colleagues what consequences can be expected from various courses of action, what the state of life will be for persons with various diseases, what the prospects for the development of a patient will be if it is given certain treatment, and so forth.[46] The value questions emerge with reference to specific diseases, or specific proposals for experimentation. Suffice it to note that theology is not medical science, and that if theology is to make any contribution to medical ethics, the theologian must not only be informed by moral philosophy but also by physicians and investigators in the area of biology.[47]

Epilogue

I have not sought to judge what the significance of theology's contribution to medical ethics is. The contribution will be of different significance to different persons, with different interests and purposes. For most persons involved in medical care and practice, the contribution of theology is likely to be of minimal importance, for the moral principles and values needed can be justified without reference to God, and the attitudes that religious beliefs ground can be grounded in other ways. From the standpoint of immediate praticality, the contribution of theology is not great, either in its extent or in its importance.

It is possible, however, to draw inferences from various medical practices and from various forms of medical ethics to make clear what basic presuppositions are operative about "being" and about "value," and about the human conditions of knowing and judging. Functional equivalents of theology are present in the patterns of action and the ethical thought of persons who find theology to be a meaningless intellectual enterprise. Perhaps the exercise of this lecture can suggest some ways in which such equivalents can be located; it would be presumptuous, however, to claim that all physicians and investigators or all authors of medical ethics have "theologies."

As was indicated, my conviction is that theology as an intellectual discipline operates within the religious consciousness, and refers to an ultimate power standing over against as well as sustaining the creation. The significance of theology's contribution to medical ethics is likely to be greatest for those who share in that religious consciousness, who have an experience of the reality of God. For them, insofar as God is the object of ultimate loyalty and ultimate obligation, it is important to clarify the relationships of religious beliefs for crucial areas of human action such as medical research and care.

Footnotes

1.   Paul Ramsey has been consistently forthright in indicating that he works out of Biblical and Christian presuppositions. "At crucial points in the analysis of medical ethics, I shall not be embarrassed to use as an interpretative principle the Biblical norm of *fidelity to covenant*, with the meaning it gives to righteousness between man and man." Paul Ramsey, *The Patient as Person*, New Haven: Yale Univ. Press, 1970, p. xii. "I always write as the ethicist I am, namely, a Christian ethicist, and not as some hypothetical common denominator." Paul Ramsey, "The Indignity of 'Death with Dignity'", *The Hastings Center Studies*, Vol. 2, No. 2, (May, 1974), p. 56.

2.   Some of the views I have in mind here are the following. "Being religious is being unconditionally concerned, whether this concern expresses itself in secular or (in the narrower sense) religious forms." Paul Tillich, *The Protestant Era*, Chicago: Univ. of Chicago Press, 1948, p. xv. "Within the world view a domain of meaning can become articulated that deserves to be called religious. This domain consists of symbols which represent an essential 'structural' trait of the world view as a whole—to wit, its inner hierarchy of significance." Thomas Luckman, *The Invisible Religion*, New York: Macmillan, 1967, p. 56. " ... A religion ... always signifies a special body of beliefs and practices having some kind of institutional organization, loose or tight. In contrast, the adjective "religious" denotes nothing in the way of a specifiable entity, either institutional or as a system of beliefs ... It denotes attitudes that may be taken toward every object and every proposed end or ideal." John Dewey, *A Common Faith*, New Haven: Yale Univ. Press, 1934, pp. 9-10. "The formula I shall expand and discuss is: a religious interest is an interest in something more important than anything else in the universe." William A. Christian, *Meaning and Truth in Religion*, Princeton, Princeton Univ. Press, 1964, p. 60. There are important

similarities between what I mean by religious dimensions of experience and the usages in the different quotations above. Luther's exposition of the first commandment makes the distinction I have in mind more dramatically, however, than I would make it: "A god is that to which we look for all good and in which we find refuge in every time of need. To have a god is nothing else than to trust and believe him with our whole heart. As I have often said, the trust and faith of the heart alone make both God and an idol." From Martin Luther, "The Large Catechism," Theodore G. Tappert, trans. and ed., *The Book of Concord*, Philadelphia: Muhlenberg Press, 1959,· p. 365. From Luther's perspective (as from Tillich's) there is a way of distinguishing between an "idol" and "God." I am concerned to indicate that one can have attitudes that function "religiously", but that the term religion is properly reserved for a relation to an ultimate power.

3. "We ought to say that a man is not really religious unless he feels that some power is bearing down on him, unless, that is, he believes he must do something about divine powers who have done something about him." Julian N. Hartt, *A Christian Critique of American Culture*, New York: Harper and Row 1967, p. 52. "Religion arises as human reaction and answer to the state of being affected totally." Richard R. Niebuhr, *Experiential Religion*, New York: Harper and Row, 1972, p. 34.

4. "If, however, we deny that there can be no absolutely immediate experience that is also meaningful, it follows that any supposed experience of God would have to be mediated in some way. Expressed in different language, every alleged experience of God would also be experience of something else at the same time. If this is so, no singular experience would stand in analogy with a sensible experience of an object as evidence that God exists. From this, however, it does not follow that a divine reality may not be ingredient in human experience in the sense that there are mediating elements in existence that will disclose the pres-

ence of God." John E. Smith, *Experience and God*, New York: Oxford Univ. Press, 1968, p. 52.

5.   Exodus 3:14a, and Exodus 3:6 and elsewhere.

6.   I have developed my views on this matter more fully in James M. Gustafson, *Can Ethics be Christian?*, Chicago: Univ. of Chicago Press, 1975, particularly in Chapter 3, "Christian Faith and 'The Sort of Person' One Becomes," and Chapter 4, "Christian Faith and the Reasons of Mind and Heart for Being Moral." In the latter chapter I have taken the experiential senses of radical dependence, gratitude, repentance, obligation, possibility and direction, as bases for indicating how the religious dimensions of experience are related to the moral dimensions.

7.   For example, in the Pentateuch, "The Lord said to Moses, 'Say to the people of Israel...'" Lev. 20:1, and throughout. Mediation through the moral order of creation can be cited whenever the "natural law" is set in a theological substructure or framework as in the work of Thomas Aquinas.

8.   For example, "The command of God as it is given to us at each moment is always and only one possibility in every conceivable particularity of its inner and outer modality. It is always a single decision, including all the thoughts and words and movements in which we execute it." Karl Barth, *Church Dogmatics*, II/2, Edinburgh: T. and T. Clark, 1957, p. 663.

9.   For example, "The interpretation of God's action in this war as redemptive and vicarious, absolute and unified judgment leads to certain consequences for human action." H. Richard Niebuhr, "War as the Judgment of God," *The Christian Century*, Vol. 60 (1943), p. 630.

10.   Kai Nielsen, "Some Remarks on the Independence of Morality from Religion," in Ian T. Ramsey, ed., *Christian Ethics and Contemporary Philosophy*, New York: Macmillan, 1966, p. 144. The quotation continues, indicating the basic argument that Nielsen is making (for a different purpose that I have here): "and if it is a moral utterance as well, it obviously does not license us

to say that any moral beliefs at all are based on religion."

11. See Gustafson, *Can Ethics be Christian?* Chap. 4, for the ways in which I argue for plausibility of such statements as these.

12. Here I am following a general line of Protestant theology which is marked by the work of Kierkegaard, *The Concept of Dread,* Princeton: Princeton Univ. Press, 1944. Reinhold Niebuhr, *The Nature and Destiny of Man,* Vol. I, New York: Scribners, 1941, Chaps. 6-9; and Paul Tillich, *The Courage to Be,* London: Nisbet and Co., 1952, especially Chap. 2.

13. A vast literature in moral philosophy is devoted to arguing that the moral point of view is the "reasonable" point of view. For some philosophers, the reasons one gives ought to be moral rather than non-moral. To give a theological reason is, in the eyes of some philosophers not only to give a "non-moral" reason for being moral, but is also mistakenly to retrieve for the argument a basis that has either a particular historical authority (and thus cannot be accepted by "all rational persons") or a dimension of experience (the religious) that is not fully rational. Arguments justifying a theological moral point of view would be made differently by different theologians. A "natural" theologian, for example, could argue that a Supreme Being is a necessary condition for any morality, both as its ontological ground and as its moral ground; indeed, a natural theologian would make a rational case for the ultimate unity of the ontological and the moral in the being (or becoming) of God. A radically confessional theologian influenced by "historicist" modes of thought might argue that all "rationality" is imbedded in historical conditions, and that the rationality of the moral philosopher is not freed from particular historical conditions and commitments. He or she might go on to argue that there are reasons, both of heart and mind, to adopt a particular moral point of view that is grounded in a religious tradition. An existentialist theologian might emphasize that "decision is king"

even for the moral philosopher, that he or she has chosen a life option. Or such a person might argue that moral choices are never fully rationally justifiable, but entail the risks involved in radical freedom in particular circumstances. My own justification, which cannot be developed here, would be a mixed argument involving some elements of each of the three "types" indicated.

14. The extension of the use of the concept of the common good that I propose can be seen more clearly by looking at a very good discussion of it in political philosophy. In his excellent essay, "Political Justice," my distinguished colleague Alan Gewirth writes, "Viewed from a social point of view, common goods may be distinguished into three groups, consisting in the necessary conditions (1) for the preservation of any society, (2) for the preservation of the distinctive sociopolitical values of a specific kind of society, and (3) for extending or advancing these values." Gewirth, "Political Justice," in Richard B. Brandt, ed., *Social Justice,* Englewood Cliffs, N.J.: Prentice-Hall, 1962, p. 165. Note that it is a "society" that is to be preserved. This at least illustrates the common context for discussion of the common good; it is the context of social and political philosophy. I am proposing that the context be extended to "nature" of which societies are part.

15. Roman Catholic readers are acquainted with the use of the "principle of totality" in medical moral theology. It was developed particularly by Pius XII, who supported certain medical experiments on the basis that the physical organism could be subordinated to the "spiritual finality of the person." For a recent discussion, see Martin Nolan, "The Principle of Totality in Moral Theology," in Charles E. Curran, ed., *Absolutes in Moral Theology?,* Washington: Corpus Books, 1968, pp. 232-48. My proposal clearly extends beyond what Pius XII and the Catholic tradition would deem to be permissible.

16. Psalm 8, which has quite properly been heard as a hymn to the wonders of human life (particularly thou

"dost crown him with glory and honor") can also be heard as a mandate to human accountability for other aspects of creation. "Thou hast given him dominion over the works of thy hands; thou hast put all things under his feet . . . " To be made "little less than God" is to have the highest degree of accountability for the well-being of the creation.

17.   I have in mind the following texts. Edwin F. Healy, S.J., *Medical Ethics*, Chicago: Loyola Univ. Press, 1956; John P. Kenny, O.P., *Principles of Medical Ethics*, 2nd ed., Westminster, Md.; Newman Press 1961; Charles J. McFadden, O.S.A., *Medical Ethics*, 4th ed., Philadelphia: F. A. Davis, 1958; Thomas G. O'Donnell, S.J., *Morals in Medicine*, 2nd ed., Westminster, Md.: Newman Press, 1959.

18.   It must be noted that natural law ethics does not necessarily lead to such restrictive rules of action as some of the texts in Roman Catholic medical ethics have prescribed. I wish to indicate that in order to have the possibility for an extension and development of natural law ethics certain basically philosophical and perhaps even theological grounds must be developed in a different way than has been the case. A number of the essays in Curran, ed., *Absolutes in Moral Theology?* properly accuse more conservative authors of having a "physicalist" bias that does not adequately take into account the distinctiveness of the nature of persons, and on this basis open possibilities for extension and revision. See also, Bruno Schüller, S. J., "Wieweit kann die Moral theologie das Naturrecht entbehren?," *Lebendiges Zeugnis*, Vol. 1 (1965), pp. 1-25, Richard A. McCormick, S. J., "Human Significance and Christian Significance," in Gene H. Outka and Paul Ramsey, eds., *Norm and Context in Christian Ethics*, New York: Scribners, 1968, pp. 233-61; and Bernard Haring, "Dynamism and continuity in a Personalistic Approach to Natural Law," in *ibid.*, pp. 199-218. Strong arguments can be made in favor of interpreting the texts in Thomas Aquinas in a more developmental way than do the authors of the medical ethics texts referred

to above.

19. Paul Ramsey, *Basic Christian Ethics*, New York: Scribners, 1950, p. 116. This position, stated in Ramsey's first book, though not consistently held in that text in my judgment, continues and is developed in his subsequent writings. Roman Catholics who are favorably disposed to Ramsey's practical judgments on medical issues have not noted sufficiently the profound theological and ethical differences between his position and theirs.

20. An excellent example of Ramsey's cogent criticism of developing medical ethics in this way is found in "Screening: An Ethicist's View," in B. Hilton, D. Callahan, M. Harris et al., eds., *Ethical Issues in Human Genetics*, New York: Plenum Press, 1973, pp. 147-60. One of the most careful efforts that has been made conceptually to deal with consequences while avoiding the pitfalls of utilitarianism is Richard A. McCormick, S.J., *Ambiguity in Moral Choice*, The 1973 Pere Marquette Theology Lecture.

21. See, for example, in Ramsey, "Screening," his discussion of amniocentesis, pp. 151-56. This procedure for the screening of the unborn he judges to be "ethically most problematic, if indeed, it is not to be morally censured" (p. 148). Basically, he argues that as long as there is no absolutely unambiguous evidence that the procedure is of no harm to the fetus, no possible benefits to the fetus or to the family can be claimed as sufficient grounds for engaging in it.

22. I recognize that in this lecture I am not addressing adequately the most substantive value issue, namely what constitutes that "well-being" of individuals and of the creation. Consistent with the views developed here, however, is the position that a process of development and discovery is also involved in that normative question. This process is necessitated principally on two bases: a) human finitude with its limitations of knowledge and understanding does not permit the certitude that we long and strive for to be realized in our efforts to disclose what "well-being" consists of,

and certainly not in a univocal or non-temporal, or simple way; and b) both natural and historical-cultural development require a process of discovery and development in our conceptualization of "well-being." Certain conditions require the alteration of at least the practical ordering of values; for example, in certain conditions the value of survival can be judged to override certain other values and rights. See "What is the Normatively Human?", in Gustafson, *Theology and Christian Ethics*, Philadelphia: Pilgrim Press, 1974, pp. 229-44, for one discussion of my views on this matter.

23. Karl Rahner, *Theological Investigations*, IX, New York: Herder and Herder, 1972, p. 224. Paul Ramsey has criticized this article severely. Ramsey remarks, "This sounds remarkably like a priestly blessing over everything, doing duty for ethics." ". . . [Rahner] clings to the belief that men are wise enough to invent themselves." "He calls for 'possible guidelines for man's self-creation, which will always remain a venture into the unforeseeable.' But Rahner gives no account of this set framework, nor does he adumbrate these laws or guidelines for man's self-creation, or attempt to say what sort of future self-direction of mankind would be worthy and what would be unworthy of man's absolute future." Paul Ramsey, *Fabricated Man*, New Haven: Yale University Press, 1970, quotations from pp. 138-40, p. 140, and pp. 141-42. While it is possible to make these judgments on the basis of a superficial reading of Rahner's article, it is clear that Ramsey does not understand the technicalities of Rahner's anthropology which render the openness possible but also put certain restrictions upon it. Although Ramsey cites the article from the German edition, he apparently did not read the article subsequent to it, "The Problem of Genetic Manipulation." If he had read that, he would have found Rahner arguing on the basis of his philosophy and theology against artificial insemination by non-husband donors, a conclusion with which Ramsey agrees. See Rahner, *Theological Investigations*, IX, pp. 225-52.

24.   Rahner, "Experiment," p.211.

25.   *Ibid.*, p. 219.

26.   *Ibid.*, p. 222.

27.   This sketch of Rahner's work is too brief and too broad to articulate the complexities of his fundamental thought as a basis for his moral point of view. In this, as in all my work on Rahner, I have been informed deeply by a decade of association with James F. Bresnahan, S.J. See, Bresnahan, "The Methodology of 'Natural Law' Ethical Reasoning in the Theology of Karl Rahner . . .", Ph.D. Diss., Yale University, 1972.

28.   Another group of theologians could be discussed in connection with the elaboration of this fifth characteristic, namely some Lutheran and biblically oriented ones. They make a distinction between "orders of creation" and "creative and ordering activity" of God. The latter opens the possibility to a developmental view of ethics. For example, "God was not active only when the world of men came into being, so that what we have now to deal with are the end-products of His original Creation. But when we move and breathe we are in a living relationship to the Creator whose work is still continuing." Gustaf Wingren, *Creation and Law.* Philadephia: Muhlenberg Press, 1961, p. 47. ". . . Man is used by the Creator as the object of His continuing work of Creation." *Ibid.* The emphasis on "God's continuing creation" could be the theological basis for an ethics which develops "law" in the course of biological and historical-cultural change. Since no theologian working from such an interpretation of Biblical theology has developed ethics with reference to medical research and care, I do not discuss this possibility further.

29.   Indeed, various "unitarianisms" in theology become authorizations for coordinated "unitarianisms" in ethics. If God is love, and only love, then love becomes the theologically grounded attitude and love becomes the principle or value of theologically grounded ethics. If God is only engaged in "liberating activity," then liberation becomes the exclusive end to be

achieved by those responding to his activity. Such unitarianisms are too simple for the richness of the human experience of the reality of God, for the convictions and statements that have been formulated from that experience, and for the complexity of moral life. The consequences of such are often perilous.

30. For a more elaborate exposition of this, see Gustafson, *Can Ethics be Christian?*, pp. 94-103.

31. Karl Barth, *Church Dogmatics*, III/4, Edinburgh: T. and T. Clark, 1961, pp. 350-51.

32. *Ibid.*, pp. 354-55.

33. *Ibid.* p. 342.

34. The bumper sticker, "Respect Life" is loaded with ambiguities and thus indicates the difficulties of commending only an attitude. In the present American context, the intention of the slogan is to marshall forces against current liberal abortion laws. But an attitude does not necessarily yield a single moral principle or support a single civil law. To "respect life" might be to respect the lives of others in addition to that of a fetus, and even if physical life is the condition *sine qua non* for other values, it is not, in the view developed here, of absolute value. "Life" as an object due respect can be highly restrictive or very inclusive; respect for life is respect for what is *valued* about life for this generation and for future generations. The slogan could well be the basis for ecological ethics as well as for legal issues on abortion.

35. For example, in northern Sweden during July, 1971, a truck driver trapped in his burning cab as a result of an accident, and bound to suffer the pain of death by burning, was killed by his associate at the driver's request. Public discussion of this incident indicated that the dominant opinion supported the associate's action, or at least would not condemn it, on the basis of the "respect" expressed for the driver's wishes.

36. See Paul Ramsey, *The Patient as Person*, pp. 117-18, 258-59, and 274-75.

37. For a discussion of this matter in the Jewish

tradition, see L. Jacobs, "Greater Love Hath No Man... The Jewish Point of View of Self-Sacrifice," *Judaism*, 6 (1957), pp. 41-47.

38.   My distinguished colleague, Edward Shils, for example, grounds the "sanctity of life" in human experience. "Is human life really sacred?," he asks. "I answer that it is, self-evidently. Its sacredness is the most primordial of experiences..." Shils, in Daniel H. Labby, ed., *Life and Death: Ethics and Options*, Seattle: University of Washington Press, 1968, pp. 18-19. I reserve the term sacred only for God.

39.   This openness is grounded in other theological affirmations as well. One important doctrine which could be explicated here is the doctrine of grace. Two aspects of the graciousness of the ultimate power are important. The first is his graciousness in creation, and in continuing creativity and development. An explication of this involves a development of views of providence and eschatology in a full theology for ethics. There are no current empirical evidences and no extrapolations toward the future which guarantee that human errors cannot cumulatively destroy the creation as we know it any more than there are evidences that the energy of the sun will be renewed when it proceeds to be exhausted; nonetheless there are religious experiential grounds for believing that created life as we know it and as future generations can know it is graced for benefits. Humans have special responsibility to insure this. The second is God's graciousness in his mercy. While surely the consequences of some human actions are more deleterious than those of others, and thus moral accountability can be "graded" to some degree with references to these, nonetheless God proffers forgiveness to all. There are powers of personal renewal to revive and re-orient persons who make grievous moral mistakes.

40.   For more extensive development of this point, see Gustafson, *Can Ethics be Christian?*, p. 98, and pp. 103-106.

41.   "Because of a remote but possible hazard to

society, a group of molecular biologists sponsored by the National Academy of Sciences (NAS) has called for a temporary ban on certain kinds of experiments that involve the genetic manipulation of living cells and viruses. This is believed to be the first time, at least in the recent history of biology, that scientists have been willing to accept any restrictions on their freedom to research, other than those to do with human experimentation." Nicholas Wade, "Genetic Manipulation: Temporary Embargo Proposed on Research," *Science*, Vol. 185 (26 July 1974), p. 332.

42. The self-criticism required by the absence of absolute certitude is applicable not only to the physicians and investigators who are the agents in interventions, but also to moralists who make judgments about those interventions. The task of the moral theologian and the moral philosopher is to provide bases for making judgments and directing actions that are generalizable if not universalizable. Uncertainty does not lead to moral chaos; indeed, the rational enterprise of ethics has as its practical end the limitation of uncertainty by providing reliable bases for judgments and actions. The aspiration to find principles and values about which all rational persons can agree is a proper one; without it surely there would be greater uncertainty than now exists. I have come to doubt, however, that the aspiration can be fulfilled by finite persons not only because there are commitments to values which involve more than rational aspects of human life, but also because finite humans can never perfectly know what constitutes the well-being of particular individuals and the whole of creation, and because that well-being itself requires different actions in particular states of the development of the creation. The moralist who judges the actions of others must also be self-critical.

43. See Joseph Fletcher, *Situation Ethics*, Philadelphia: Westminster Press, 1966. William K. Frankena classes Fletcher as a utilitarian; see Frankena, *Ethics*, 2nd ed., Englewood-Cliffs: Prentice-Hall,

1973, p. 36 and pp. 55-56. For an example of Fletcher's ethical theory applied to genetics, see Fletcher, "Ethical Aspects of Genetic Controls," in *New England Journal of Medicine*, Vol. 285 (1971), pp. 776-83.

44. See John Rawls, "Two Concepts of Rules," reprinted in Philippa Foot, ed., *Theories of Ethics*, Oxford: Oxford Univ. Press, 1967, pp. 144-70. The article develops other distinctions which have influenced the way in which the rest of this lecture has been developed, though I do not cite it more.

45. For Barth's special ethics, see *Church Dogmatics*, III/4; especially relevant here is the section on the "Protection of Life," pp. 397-470. "However dangerous it might sound in relation to all that has been said thus far, it must also be said that in faith, and in a vicarious intercessory faith for others too, there is a forgiveness which can be appropriated even for this sin, even for the great modern sin of abortion," p. 419. "Let us be quite frank and say that there are situations in which the killing of germinating life does not constitute murder but is in fact commanded," p. 421. For Barth's discussion of euthanasia, see pp. 423-27.

46. For an example of how ethical reflection must take into account specific diseases even within the general class of genetic diseases, see Gustafson, "Genetic Screening and Human Values," in Daniel Bergsma, ed., *Ethical, Social and Legal Dimensions of Screening for Human Genetic Disease*, New York: Stratton International Medical Book Corp., 1974, pp. 203-10.

47. An earlier draft of this lecture was read at Georgetown University, November 4, 1974, under the auspices of the Department of Philosophy and the Kennedy Center for Bioethics. I wish to acknowledge the benefits I received from the oral discussion at that time, and particularly from subsequent written communications from Professor Henry B. Veatch and Dr. Leon R. Kass.

The Père Marquette Lectures in Theology

1991 *Faith, History and Cultures: Stability and Change in Church Teachings*
    Walter H. Principe, C.S.B.
    University of Toronto

1992 *Universe and Creed*
    Stanley L. Jaki
    Seton Hall University

1993 *The Resurrection of Jesus Christ: Some Contemporary Issues*
    Gerald G. O'Collins, S.J.
    Gregorian Pontifical University

1994 *Seeking God in Contemporary Culture*
    Most Reverend Rembert G. Weakland, O.S.B.
    Archbishop of Milwaukee

1995 *The Book of Proverbs and Our Search for Wisdom*
    Richard J. Clifford, S.J.
    Weston Jesuit School of Theology

1996 *Orthodox and Catholic Sister Churches: East is West and West is East*
    Michael A. Fahey, S.J.
    University of St. Michael's College, Toronto

1997 *'Faith Adoring the Mystery': Reading the Bible with St. Ephræm the Syrian*
    Sidney H. Griffith
    Catholic University of America

1998 *Is There Life after Death?*
    Jürgen Moltmann
    Eberhard-Karls Universität
    Tübingen, Germany

1999 *Moral Theology at the End of the Century*
    Charles E. Curran
    Elizabeth Scurlock University Professor of Human Values
    Southern Methodist University

2000 *Is the Reformation over?*
    Geoffrey Wainwright

2001 *In Procession before the World: Martyrdom As Public Liturgy in Early Christianity*
    Robin Darling Young

About the Père Marquette Lecture Series
The Annual Père Marquette Lecture Series began at Marquette University in the Spring of 1969. Ideal for classroom use, library additions, or private collections, the Père Marquette Lecture Series has received international acceptance by scholars, universities, and libraries. Hardbound in blue cloth with gold stamped covers. Uniform style and price ($15 each). Some reprints with soft covers. Regular reprinting keeps all volumes available. Ordering information (purchase orders, checks, and major credit cards accepted):

Marquette University Press
  1444 U.S. Route 42
  P.O. Box 388
  Ashland OH 44903

  Order Toll-Free (800) 247-6553
  fax: (419) 281 6883

Editorial Address:
  Dr. Andrew Tallon, Director
  Marquette University Press
  Box 1881
  Milwaukee WI 53201-1881

phone:	(414) 288-7298
fax:	(414) 288-3300
internet:	andrew.tallon@marquette.edu
web:	www.marquette.edu/mupress/